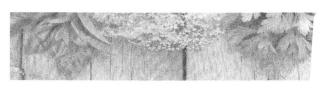

NATURAL HOME REMEDIES

FOR ALL

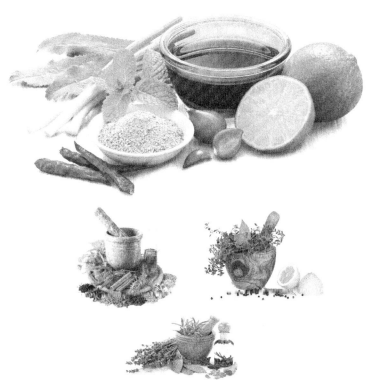

BY
HAKEEM MOULANA JALEEL MUHAMMAD PANDOR

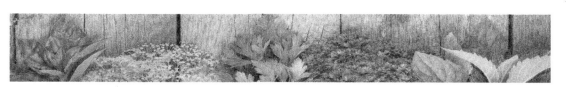

Prepared by: Jamiatul Ulama (KZN)
Ta'limi Board
4 Third Avenue
P.O.Box 26024
Isipingo Beach
4115
South Africa

Natural Home Remedies

Contents

- 7 Guidelines for Good Health 6
- Important ingredients and plants to be kept and grown at home 10
- Sure Prescription for any ailment 11
- Acid Reflux / Heart Burn 12
  - Stomach pain Acid reflux / Heart burn 12
- Acne 12
- Arthritis 13
- Asthma 15
- Bad Breath 16
  - Remedy: 2 16
- Bladder 17
  - Weak Bladder 17
- Bedsores 17
  - Remedy: 2 17
- Blood Clot 17
- Body Pains 18
  - Remedy: 2 18
  - Remedy: 3 18
  - Body Pains 19
  - Remedy: 5 19
  - Joints Pains 19
  - Bone Pains 19
- Boils 20
  - Boil on Eye (Aanfede) 21
- Bronchitis 21
- Burns 22
- Cold/ Running Nose 22
  - Inhaling steam vapours 24
  - Ginger Tea (for colds & Flu) 26

Natural Home Remedies

Constipation 27
    Faakee 27

Cough 28
    (Phlegmy cough) 29
    (Dry cough) 29
    (Also used for cold, reducing fever and upset stomach) 29
        Cough Mixture 32
        (For eliminating coughs) 33

Cuts & Wounds 33
Dandruff 34
Dehydration 34
Dental Care 35
    (Toothache) 35

Detox 35
Diabetes 36
Diarrhoea 37
Dizziness 38
Ear-ache 38
Energy 38
    (Energy for the entire day) 38

Eyesight 39
Feet 39
    Swollen Feet 39

Fever 39
Flu 40
Gout 41
    Maintenance treatment for gout 41

Headache 42
    Headache caused through nose congestion 42
    Migraine headaches 43

Natural Home Remedies

- Heart Disease / Cholesterol 43
  - Palpitations & short breadth 44
    - Mint tea 45
    - Barley Water 45
- Hiccups 46
- Intestines 46
- Indigestion 47
- Jaundice 47
- Kidney Stones 48
- Massage Oil 48
- Memory 49
- Mouth sores 49
- Nausea 50
- Nose Bleeding 50
- Phlegm 51
- Piles 51
- Pressure 52
  - (Low pressure) 52
  - (High Pressure) 52
- Psoriasis 53
- Rash 54
- Rejuvenate 54
- Ringworms 54
- Sprain 55
- Stings 55
- Stomach Pain 56
- Strength 56
- Stroke 57
- Throat 57
  - (Swelling of the throat) 57
  - (Laryngitis - inflammation of voice box) 57

(Sore throat)	58
Ulcers	59
(For bleeding ulcer)	59
Vomiting & Phlegm	60
Warts	60
Wheezing	60
BABIES AND MOTHERS	61
For Colic Babies	61
Balm to rub on chest for children with Colds	62
Infants Cold	62
Mixture to increase Breastmilk	62
Confinement Medication	63
After Birth	63
Kahyo	63
3 O'clock porridge masala	65
Hoowa (soowa/anise) Sook Mookh	65
Kwaar paak	66
Methi paak	67
Menstruation - For pain	68
For heavy bleeding	68
For weakness: during confinement and periods	69
Post Natal Care	69
Herbal bath	69
General Guidelines for Health in winter	70
Terminology	71

Natural Home Remedies

بِسْمِ اللهِ الرَّحْمٰنِ الرَّحِيْمِ

Foreword

نحمده ونصلى على رسوله الكريم ، اما بعد

I have perused this booklet in your hands and have found it to be very useful. Marhoom Hakeem Yusuf Molvi (rahimahullah) used to always tell me, "Listen to the wisdom of the old people and you will acquire knowledge which is not found even in books." There is an Arabic saying as well,

سَلِ الْمُجَرَّبْ وَلَا تَسْئَلِ الْحَكِيْم

"Ask the experienced person *and not the philosopher.*"

This book is full of tried and tested recipes which have been found useful. Here I have to sound a note of caution that if one is not sure of any ingredient helping them and it might be harmful for them, then it should be queried from a qualified Hakeem. Secondly, if no benefit is noticed, then too a Hakeem has to be consulted. It will help a person tremendously to help themselves recover using natural methods instead of going through conventional medication which is really costly and full of harmful side effects.

I ask Allah to accept this work and make it beneficial to the Ummah. *Aameen.*

Hakeem Moulana Jaleel Muhammad Pandor

7 Guidelines for Good Health

"Verily your body has a right over you." (Hadith)

Rasulullah (Sallallahu alayhi Wasallam) has mentioned that there are two favours which most people take lightly; "Good health and free time." Looking after our health is an essential part of a Muslim's life. If we are not careful regarding this important aspect of our lives, then we may be deprived of many important aamaal (May Allah Ta'ala protect us all). We may be unable to perform Salaah with Jama'ah, go out in the path of Allah, make Jihaad and help the poor and needy if we do not preserve good health.

In another Hadith, Rasulullah (Sallallahu alayhi Wasallam) has mentioned, "A strong Muslim is better and more beloved to Allah Ta'ala than a weak Muslim."

We have been repeatedly taught in the Ahaadith to make dua for good health and seek Allah Ta'ala's protection from dreadful diseases. One such dua is as follows, "O Allah! Keep my hearing well, keep my sight well and keep my body well."

Make shukar and thank Allah Ta'ala for the good health that we enjoy and in turn Allah Ta'ala will increase us in good health.

Health and sickness are both from Allah Ta'ala alone. However, we have been commanded in the Qur'aan to take precautions. If we adhere to the following 7 points, Insha Allah, we will enjoy good health throughout our lives.

Natural Home Remedies

1. Clean Air

Make a point of breathing in fresh clean air. After Fajr, take a walk and breathe in deeply from your nose allowing the fresh morning air to filter through your lungs. Exhale from your mouth. Hadhrat Molana Hakeem Muhammad Akhtar Saahib (Rahimahullah) has mentioned, "Subah ki hawa, Laakho ki dawa" (The fresh morning air is a medicine for hundreds of thousands of ailments).

Allow fresh air and sunlight into the home daily and ensure that the house is free from dampness.

Hadhrat Moulana Ashraf Ali Thaanwi (rahmatullahi alayh) used to say that if a person takes a walk after the Fajr Salaah with the intention of enjoying good health, then he will Insha Allah receive the same reward as the one who sat in the masjid up to Ishraaq Salaah.

Refrain totally from smoking or sitting near those who smoke.

2. Clean Water

Drink clean fresh water. If possible, drink rain water or borehole water (provided it is tested and declared safe to drink). If this is not available, install a water purifying unit in your home whereby you can obtain filtered water instead of the water directly from the tap. Do ensure that you use a good quality filter,

Drink 8 glasss (+- 2 litres) of water per day.
Avoid drinking water ½ an hour before and after meals.
Try and avoid drinking very cold or iced water.

3. Exercise

Most of us are unmindful of this. One should exercise at least 3 times a week for 20-30 minutes.

People with busy schedules may suffice with at least 15 press-ups and 20 sit-ups at the beginning of the day.

At the least, a brisk walk every second day for approximately 20 minutes will do you much good. Those men who live within walking distance from the masjid should make it a habit to walk to the masjid for their five times Salaah. (NB. Women should not go out walking on the street. Rather they should walk in their homes or in their yards).

4. Balanced diet

Eat two meals a day instead of three. Supper should be a light meal. Refrain from eating processed foods (polonies, sausages, patties, foods with artificial flavouring, colouring, msg, preservatives, etc.).
Avoid eating too much of oily foods or food fried in oil.
Avoid eating between meals.

Don't overeat. We learn from the Hadith of Rasulullah (Sallallahu alayhi Wasallam) to reserve one third of the stomach for food, one third for water and one third for air.

Cook simple meals. Avoid cooking too many varieties for one meal. The Hakeems are of the opinion that eating various different types of food in one meal is not conducive to good health.

5. Sleep

Hadhrat Moulana In'aamul Hasan Saahib (Rahimahullah) had advised that every person should get 6 hours of sound sleep daily. One cannot function efficiently without having sufficient sleep.

Rasulullah (Sallallahu alayhi Wasallam) has encouraged us to have an afternoon nap (+- 45 minutes). This sleep in medical terms is referred to as a power nap. Nabi (Sallallahu alayhi Wasallam), has said that having an afternoon nap will assist one in waking up for the Tahajjud Salaah.

6. Control of emotions

Rasulullah (Sallallahu alayhi Wasallam), has, on several occasions, cautioned the ummat about controlling their emotions. There are many Ahaadith of Nabi (Sallallahu alayhi Wasallam) wherein there are severe warnings for those who do not control their anger as well as those who harbour jealousy, hatred and rancour in their hearts for others. This eventually builds into stress within us. Stress has become very common. Due to our hectic lifestyles, the long hours that we work, we begin to stress and those around us suffer the consequences.

People who cannot manage their stress levels adequately are prone to cardiovascular high blood pressure, diabetes and other illnesses.

7. Elimination of toxins (Detox)

Due to our unhealthy diet, we have a build-up of toxins in our bodies. These toxins need to be eliminated from time to time. Toxin build-up in the colon is the beginning of many illnesses.
In order to eliminate these toxins, one should take 2 Tablespoons of Castor oil in half a glass of orange juice every two months.
Drinking a lot of water also helps to eliminate toxins from the body.
May Allah Ta'ala keep us all physically and spiritually healthy. Aameen.

Important ingredients and plants to be kept and grown at home

Ingredients:

1. Bicarbonate of soda
2. Nutmeg
3. Apple Cider Vinegar
4. Turmeric Powder (arad)
5. Epsom Salt
6. Codliver Oil
7. Methi (fenugreek)
8. Ginger Powder
9. Ajmo (tymol / caraway seeds)
10. Maizena
11. Olive Oil
12. Elachi (cardamom)
13. Ispaghula
14. Khus Khus (poppy seeds)
15. Honey

Plants:

1. Aloe
2. lavender
3. Fudina (Mint)
4. Lemon Grass
5. Thyme
6. Curry leaves
7. Celery
8. Spring Onion

Sure Prescription for any ailment

In case of any illness, a person should first adopt the following steps before taking any medication.

- Perform 2 Rakaats of Salaatul Haajah.
- Make earnest Dua to Allah to grant you Shifaa.
- Give some Sadaqah daily.
- Increase the recitation of Istighfaar.
- Read Surah Faatihah 7 times. Blow in the water and drink. Also blow on the sick patient.
- Do this with complete Yaqeen (conviction) in the words of Allah Ta'ala and Nabi Muhammad (sallallahu alayhi wasallam).
- First resort to some home remedy.
- Thereafter, if medical help is required, one may do so.

Acid Reflux / Heart Burn

Remedy: 1

- ¼ tsp B.I Soda
- ¼ cup hot water

Mix together and drink.

Remedy: 2

Stomach pain Acid reflux / Heart burn

- 1 tsp apple cider vinegar
- ½ glass water

Add 1 tsp Apple cider vinegar to ½ glass water. Sip this water while eating.

Acne

Remedy:1

- 1 litre Milk (preferably dilute with water)
- 2 tsp nutmeg (jaifal)
- Honey to sweeten

Bring milk to boil, turn down the heat and stir in the honey and nutmeg (jaifal). Simmer until the milk is reduced to half its volume. Drink 1 cup every night for 1 week. Discontinue for 2 weeks. Continue drinking 1 cup every night for another week.

Remedy: 2

- Bran
- Baking soda
- Water
- Apple cider vinegar

Make a face pack from bran, baking soda and water. Apply to the Face and leave on for 15 mins. Rinse of with apple cider vinegar and water. (one part vinegar to 8 parts water)

Note: Cut out sweet and oily foods and excessive dairy products.

Arthritis

Remedy: 1

- ½ tsp arad (haldi / turmeric powder)
- 1 ½ tsp lemon juice

Mix in warm water every morning and drink.

Remedy: 2

- 3 Tblsp fresh lemon juice
- 3 Tblsp Epsom salts
- 1 litre warm water

Mix 3 Tblsp fresh lemon juice, 3 Tblsp Epsom salts in 1 litre of warm water. Take 1 tsp morning and night.

Remedy: 3
- **3 cups Epsom salts**

Add 3 cups Epsom salt in hot bath water and soak in it. The magnesium in the salt is absorbed by the body. It soothes and relaxes stiff joints & muscles.

Remedy: 4
- **1 Tblsp cod liver oil**
- **4 Tblsp Milk**

Mix very well and take as the last thing at night on an empty stomach.

N.B - Not to be taken for more than 3 months at a time.

Remedy: 5
- **½ kg methi (fenugreek) ground**

Take 1 tsp of ground methi (fenugreek) with lukewarm water at bedtime.

Remedy: 6
- **¼ kg kulunji (black seeds) ground**
- **1 litre olive oil**

Take kulunji (black seeds) and mix with olive oil, boil for ½ hour. When cool fill in bottle. Apply when needed.

Remedy: 7
- **Sweet oil**
- **Camphor oil**
- **Bloekoem oil (eucalyptus oil)**

Mix all 3 oils, shake well and rub when needed.

Asthma

Remedy: 1

- 4 x Maree (pepper)
- 4 x Raisins (without seeds)

Chew them well first thing in the morning.

Remedy: 2

- ½ cup ajmo (tymol seeds / caraway)
- Honey

Roast till dark. When cool grind in coffee grinder. Mix 1 tsp honey and 1tsp ajmo (caraway) powder and take 2 times a day.

Remedy: 3

- 1 large onion peeled and sliced
- ½ cup brown sugar

Sprinkle ½ cup brown sugar over the sliced onions. Cover and leave overnight. Take 1 tsp twice a day.

Remedy: 4

- 1 onion
- Brown sugar
- ¼ cup lemon juice
- Honey

1 onion cut into thick slices, cover with brown sugar and leave overnight. ¼ cup lemon juice, top up with water and honey (onion will make a syrup). Add 1 Tblsp of syrup to lemon and honey water. Drink a little at a time throughout the day.

Remedy: 5

- 5 almonds soaked overnight in ¾ cup water.
- 1 tsp khus-khus (poppy seeds), soaked.
- 5 pumpkin kernels
- 1 cup warm water
- honey

Next morning skin almonds. Add 5 pumpkin kernels and grind everything together finely, add ½ cup warm milk and ¾ tsp honey.

Very good for insomnia (sleeplessness) as well.

Bad Breath

Remedy: 1

- A slice of cucumber

Place in mouth for 30 seconds to 1 min then discard in the garden.

Remedy: 2

- ½ tsp apple cider vinegar

Dilute ½ tsp apple cider vinegar in a glass of water and use for gargling (10 seconds at a time).

Bladder

Weak Bladder

Remedy: 1

- ¼ tsp ginger powder

¼ tsp ginger powder taken with water every morning.

Bedsores

Remedy: 1

- **Young & tender cabbage leaves**

Young and tender cabbage leaves which are applied to bedsores give relief from discomfort while healing.

Remedy: 2

- **Maizena**
- **ghee**

Maizena and ghee; mix and rub on tender places.

Blood Clot

Remedy: 1

- **1 clove garlic**
- **1 Tblsp olive oil**

- **1 glass of water mixed with 2 tsp honey**

Drink the above before Fajr Salaah. Also have 3 Tblsp onion juice before breakfast.

Body Pains

Remedy: 1

- **½ cup apple cider vinegar**
- **1 litre water**

Mix and massage body with water.

Remedy: 2

- **2 Tblsp fine salt (must be table salt)**
- **½ cup Epsom salt**
- **½ cup apple cider vinegar (optional)**

Dissolve above ingredients in a tub of water and sit therein for a considerable amount of time.

Remedy: 3

- **½ tsp turmeric powder**
- **½ cup water**

Have on an empty stomach in the morning.

Remedy: 4

Body Pains

- 1 tsp of turmeric (arad) powder
- 1 glass of water
- 1 tsp of honey (optional)

Mix well and drink before meals.

Remedy: 5

Joints Pains

- 250g pure honey
- ¼ cup Methi (fenugreek) powder
- 2 tsp almond powder
- 1 tsp elachi (cardamom) powder
- 2 tsp ginger powder
- 2 tsp butter ghee
- 1 tsp nutmeg (jaifal) powder

Mix everything thoroughly and put in a bottle. Dose - 1 tsp daily after breakfast for 40 days.

Remedy: 6

Bone Pains

- ½ cup methi (fenugreek) powder
- ½ cup Ajmo (tymol seeds / caraway) powder

- ¼ cup black jeeroo (cumin)

Take 1 tsp

Boils

Remedy: 1

- 2 Tblsp flour
- 2 Tblsp sugar
- 2 Tblsp olive oil
- 2 Tblsp water

Mix above ingredients and apply on affected area.

Remedy: 2

Fenugreek (methi) seeds are also an excellent blood and liver cleanser, 1. tsp of the powder should be taken in a glass of milk before sleeping.

Remedy: 3

Crush a few cloves of garlic and apply to the boil.

Remedy: 4

Make a paste with glycerine and epsom salt and warm slightly, put onto boil and tie up. (it will draw out all the matter, etc)

Remedy: 5

Take a slice of onion and attach it to the boil with a plaster. (This works wonders.)

Remedy: 6

Boil on Eye (Aanfede)

Take one clove and soak it in water, rub that water onto the eye.

Soak date pits in water and make into a paste, put on eye.

Bronchitis

Remedy: 1

- 1 loaf whole wheat bread
- Butter
- salt

Oven dry one loaf whole wheat bread. Store in an airtight container. Crumble 2 slices, boil with 1 ¼ cup water, 1 tsp butter and a pinch of salt. Strain and drink as hot as possible upon awakening and at bedtime.

Remedy: 2

- 60g finely chopped garlic
- honey

Pour 600ml boiling water over 60g finely chopped garlic. Allow to stand in a sealed container for ten (10) hours. Add enough honey to contents till a syrup forms. Take 1-2 tsp 3 times a day with meals.

Remedy: 3

- Saffron strands
- Goats milk

Saffron strands infused in boiled goats milk will give relief to a chesty person.

Burns

Remedy: 1

- **A slice of tomato**
- **Honey**
- **Egg-white**

Apply any of the above on the wound.

Remedy:

- **Flour**

Dip wound in flour for ± 5 mins to avoid blistering.

Remedy: 3

Place wound in ice-cold water.

Cold/ Running Nose

Remedy: 1

- **¼ tsp Arad (haldi / turmeric powder)**
- **¼ tsp fine salt**
- **¼ tsp B.I Soda**

Mix together with ¼ cup hot water and add honey to sweeten. Drink mixture twice a day.

Remedy 2:

- 2 Tblsp honey
- ¼ tsp black pepper
- ¼ tsp cinnamon powder
- ¼ tsp nutmeg (jaifal) powder

Squeeze ½ lemon and mix all these ingredients in a glass. Warm mixture and drink.

Remedy: 3

- ½ cup warm water
- ½ tsp salt

Mix thoroughly, put 3 drops in each nostril 2 times a day.

Remedy: 4

- 1 tsp Arad (haldi / turmeric powder)
- 1 tsp honey
- ¼ tsp elachi (cardamom)

Boil 1 cup milk and add the remaining ingredients in.

Remedy: 5

Wipe paan (betel) leaves dry. Brush olive oil on paan (betel) leaves. Make oven tray hot. Remove from oven and place 4 big paan (betel) leaves on it. Place 1 on the chest 2 on the sides, 1 on the back. Wrap with thin material and leave overnight.

Remedy: 6

Inhaling steam vapours

- **Apple cider vinegar**
- **A pinch of arad (haldi / turmeric powder) or eucalyptus oil**

Add few drops apple cider vinegar, a pinch of Arad (haldi / turmeric powder), or eucalyptus oil to steaming water and inhale. Helps loosen tight chest, clears congestion in nose and relieves headache.

Remedy: 7

Rub vicks on chest & under feet at bed time and put on socks and sleep. (Excellent for cold and coughs.)

Remedy: 8

- **Lemon juice**
- **honey**

Mix lemon juice & honey in warm water and have 3 times a day.

Remedy: 9

- **garlic cloves**
- **Salt**
- **pepper**

Boil a few cloves of garlic in water and consume this soup (add salt / pepper for taste). Take morning & evening.

Natural Home Remedies

Remedy: 10
- Ginger
- honey

Grate or crush a piece of ginger. Add it to boiling water. Sweeten with honey and drink as hot as possible. Relieves sore throat & clears the feeling of heavy headedness.

Remedy: 11
- Few pieces of ginger
- ¼ tsp arad (haldi / turmeric powder)
- 3 pepper corns
- 1/4 tsp ajmo (caraway)
- 1 elachi (cardamom)
- 1 stick cinnamon

Boil in 1 cup milk and sweeten with honey. Drink before sleeping.

Remedy: 12

Have Fruits like oranges, lemon, etc. which are high in vitamin C.

Remedy: 13

Chicken soup helps give relief from colds. Fish is also very good. Avoid red meat when feeling fluish.

Remedy: 14
- 1 tsp honey
- ½ tsp nutmeg (jaifal)
- ½ tsp lemon juice

Mix and lick as desired.

Remedy: 15

- 1 tsp wheat bran
- 5 black peppercorns
- ½ tsp salt
- 1 ½ cups water

Boil the above until ¾ cup remains then strain. This is one dose, to be taken warm and unsweetened upon awakening and at bedtime for 4-7 days.

Remedy: 16

- black pepper
- honey
- apple-cider vinegar

Make a paste and suck a little.

Remedy: 17

Ginger Tea (for colds & Flu)

- 1 tsp grated ginger
- 1 stick of cinnamon
- 1 elachi (cardamom)
- 3 cups water

Boil until 1 cup remains, sweeten with honey and drink before going to bed.

Constipation

Remedy: 1

Faakee

- 5oog soowa
- 250g ajmo
- 2 Tblsp asafoetida (heeng)
- 2 Tblsp black salt
- 75g senna leaves

Roast ajmo and soowa. When cool grind everything together in a coffee grinder. Have a teaspoon of the mixture every now and again.

Remedy: 2

Ispaghul (husk) - mixed with honey and warm water.

Remedy: 3

- 1-2 tsp somph (fennel)
- 1 cup water
- 1 cinnamon stick
- 1 tsp black jeeru (cumin)

Boil till ¾ cup water then drink.

Remedy: 4

Soak a few prunes overnight. Drink the water in the morning.

Remedy: 5

1 Tblsp olive oil every night before sleeping.

Remedy: 6
- Prunes
- Raisins
- Figs

Remedy: 7
- Warm honey water

Remedy: 8
Add 2 Tblsp apple-cider vinegar to a glass of water. Drink mixture 3x a day. The vinegar can be mixed with apple juice or grape juice to make it more palatable.

Remedy: 9
2-3 glasses of warm water an hour before breakfast.

Remedy: 10
Boil prunes in water - dried or fresh. Add 1 lemon peel and cinnamon. Strain and drink.

Cough

Remedy: 1
- ½ tsp dry ginger powder
- ¼ tsp cinnamon powder
- honey

Boil ½ teaspoon of dry ginger powder, ¼ teaspoon cinnamon powder in a cup of water. Sweeten with honey and drink twice a daily.

Remedy: 2

(Phlegmy cough)

- ½ tsp turmeric (haldi / turmeric) powder
- ¼ tsp salt
- ¼ tsp ground elachi (cardamom)
- 2 tsp honey

Mix & have 1 Tblsp morning and evening

Remedy: 3

(Dry cough)

- ½ cup olive oil
- ½ cup honey

Mix thoroughly take 1 Tblsp two times a day.

Remedy: 4

(Also used for cold, reducing fever and upset stomach)

- ½ cup ajmo (tymol seeds /caraway)

Roast till dark. When cool grind in coffee grinder. Mix 2 tsp honey and 1 tsp ajmo (caraway) powder and take 2 times a day (morning & evening).

Remedy: 5

- **1 Tblsp honey**
- **5 drops lemon juice**
- **pinch of black pepper**

Mix all ingredients and have twice a day.

Remedy: 6

- **¼ cup boiling water**
- **½ tsp salt**
- **1 tsp vinegar**
- **1 Tblsp honey.**

Mix together and drink.

Remedy: 7

- **1 cup water**
- **2 small pieces of cinnamon sticks**
- **1 whole elachi (cardamom)**
- **1 clove**

Boil the above till it becomes ¾ cup. Sweeten well with honey and drink 3 times a day.

Remedy: 8

Boil 2 tsp somph (fennel) in 2 cups water until 1 ½ cups remain. Drink ¼ cup with ½ tsp honey twice a day.

Remedy: 9

- **1 tsp butter**
- **1 tsp vinegar**

- 1 tsp honey
- ¼ cup water

Boil together and have first thing in the morning and last thing at night.

Remedy: 10

- 5 cloves
- 3 elachi (cardamom)
- 5 black pepper corns
- 1 tsp somph
- 2 pieces cinnamon sticks
- Mint leaves
- A small piece of ginger

Boil together for 5 minutes and drink a cupful with honey.

Remedy: 11

- 4 Almonds
- 1 tsp khus-khus (poppy seeds)
- 2 elachi (cardamom) seeds
- 4 tsp honey - warm

Grind almond, khus-khus (poppy seeds) + elachi (cardamom) till very fine, add to honey. ¾ tsp morning and evening.

Remedy: 12

- 1 grain rough salt

For temporary relief from cough at night, place medium sized grain of rough salt under the tongue.

N.B This will not make the cough better but it will ensure a sound sleep.

Remedy: 13

Cough Mixture

- 2kg dark brown sugar
- 1 x 750 ml bottle vinegar
- 2 x 750 ml bottles water
- pinch salt
- ½ cup apple cider vinegar
- 7 pieces thuj (cinnamon sticks)
- 11 pieces cloves
- 7 pieces whole black pepper
- 27 pieces elachi (cardamom)
- ½ cup treacle
- 1 cup honey

Grind thuj, cloves, pepper and elachi (cardamom) roughly.

Place all ingredients besides treacle and honey in a large pot.

Dissolve sugar and put to boil until mixture becomes thick like syrup.

Add treacle and honey and boil for a minute.

When cold strain and store in bottles.

N.B. Also recommended for asthma. Take 1 Tblsp at a time - every hour if cough is bad.

Remedy: 14

(For eliminating coughs)

1. Braise 1 tsp cake flour with 1 tsp butter. Add 1 cup milk and allow to boil for 1-2 minutes. Add 1 tsp honey and a pinch of salt. Drink as hot as possible.

2. Take ¼ cup boiling water; add ½ tsp butter and 1 tsp sugar, a pinch of salt and 1 tsp honey. Drink it hot.

3. Boil 1 cup milk with 3-4 strands of saffron and honey and drink before bedtime.

Remedy: 15

- **Ajmo leaf (squeezed)**
- **1 tsp honey**

Wash out a small cup with boiling water. Mix 1 tsp honey and the squeezed ajmo leaf in this cup. Give to patient. Same can be done with fudina leaves (Madina fudina).

Cuts & Wounds

Remedy: 1

- **Honey**

Apply honey to stop bleeding.

Remedy: 2

- **turmeric**

Apply turmeric powder. This acts as an antiseptic.

Dandruff

Remedy: 1

- 1 tsp lemon juice
- 1 tsp honey
- 1 tsp vinegar
- 1 tsp olive oil

Mix all ingredients and massage into scalp before bathing.

Remedy: 2

- 1 Tblsp castor oil
- 1 Tblsp bi-carb
- 1 Tblsp lemon juice

Mix all ingredients and warm. Massage into scalp 2 hours before bathing.

Dehydration

Remedy: 1

- 1 litre water
- 4 Tblsp honey (raw)
- 1 level tsp rock salt

Mix well together and drink. *8 tsp sugar can be used in place of honey.

Dental Care

Remedy: 1

Dissolve 1 tsp of honey in ½ a cup of vinegar and gargle. This helps strengthen the teeth and gums and remove stains and filth from the teeth.

(Toothache)

Remedy: 1

Apply clove oil on gums.

Remedy: 2

Take a pinch of baking powder and rub on the aching tooth.

Remedy: 3

- **21 guava leaves**

To strengthen loose teeth and bleeding gums, boil 21 guava leaves in 3 litres of water for 10 min. Cool and fill in a bottle with 5 of the leaves. Gargle 3 time a day. Can be stored for 3 weeks.

Detox

Remedy: 1

½ a glass hot water, ¼ tsp ginger powder.

Remedy:5

1 glass boiled water ½ an hour before meals 3 times a day.

Diabetes

Remedy: 1

- 1 cup lemon juice
- ½ cup garlic
- 1 onion
- 2 cups water

Liquidize lemon juice, garlic and onion. Boil with water until half remains. Strain. Keep in fridge. Drink 1-2. Tblsp every morning.

Remedy: 2

- 2 Tblsp methi (fenugreek) seeds
- 1 cup water

Boil for 10 mins. Leave overnight. Strain. Leave in fridge. Drink ¼ cup first thing in the morning.

*Very good for high sugar level in diabetes.

Remedy:3

Chew 10 curry leaves in the morning on an empty stomach for 3 months.

*Also good for obesity.

Remedy: 4

- Sugar
- Green beans
- Kulunji (black seeds)
- Garlic finely sliced
- Lemon juice

Boil in water for few minutes and eat.

Remedy: 5

Chew the leaves of the custard apple tree.

Diarrhoea

Remedy: 1

- **Roast 5 elachi (cardamom)**

Put in saucepan till black. Boil in 1 cup water and drink.

Remedy: 2

- **Apples / apple juice.**

Remedy: 3

- **Yoghurt**

Kills bacteria.

Remedy: 4

- **1 Tblsp ispaghul**
- **Rose syrup**

Take 1 glass of water, sweeten with rose syrup and add 1 Tblsp ispaghul.

Remedy: 5

- **2 Tblsp condensed milk**

Cools stomach.

Remedy: 6

- Bananas.

Dizziness

- 12g dhania (coriander) seeds - coarsely crushed
- 12g aamla powder

Soak in 200ml boiling water for 8-12 hours. 100ml morning and evenings.

Ear-ache

Remedy: 1

Pour 1 or 2 drops of warm olive oil in the ear and plug the ear with a piece of cotton wool.

Remedy: 2

Boil strong coffee and strain through a muslin cloth, add a pinch of salt. Warm slightly and put 3 drops in ear.

Energy

Remedy: I

(Energy for the entire day)

Soak 4 black raisins and 1 tsp crushed sugar candy in a glass of water overnight and drink first thing in the morning.

Eyesight

Remedy: 1

Add 250g of somph (fennel) to 500g blanched almonds. Stamp both ingredients fine. Keep in a bottle. Take 6-12g with hot milk before going to bed at night.

*To be taken For at least 3 months.

Remedy: 2

Chew curry leaves for cataract.

Feet

Swollen Feet

Remedy: 1

Swollen feet will be relieved if soaked in hot water to which vinegar has been added. A 10 min. soak will give considerable relief.

Remedy: 2

Lie down on your back with feet raised slightly above body level.

Fever

Remedy: 1

Dip a cotton hanky in a bowl of vinegar and squeeze lightly, thereafter place on the head.

Remedy: 2

Mix equal amounts coconut oil and vinegar and apply on joints.

*N.B. Do not apply on head and liver area.

Remedy: 3

If the fever is extremely severe, put some ice in a cloth and place beneath the navel.

Flu

Remedy: 1

- **1½ heaped tsp Arad (haldi / turmeric powder)**
- **Few grains of rough salt**
- **1 litre water**

Boil and drink little at a time.

Remedy: 2

- **½ cup ajmo (tymol / caraway)**

Roast till dark. When cool grind in coffee grinder. Mix 1 tsp honey and 1 tsp ajmo (caraway) powder and take 2 times a day.

Remedy: 3

- **1 Tblsp somph (fennel)**
- **1 Tblsp lemon juice**
- **½ Tblsp ginger juice**
- **1 Tblsp honey**

Boil in water. Drink 1 cup in the morning and 1 cup at night.

Gout

Remedy: 1

When you have a gout attack do as Follows; Mix 1 teaspoon bi-carbonate of soda and lemon juice from 2 lemons. Have every 2 hours till pain subsides.

Remedy: 2

- ½ bottle honey
- ¼ cup crushed methi
- 2 tsp ginger powder
- 1 tsp Nutmeg (jaifal) powder
- 1 tsp Elachi (cardamom)
- 2 tsp fine badaam (almond) powder
- 1 tsp butter ghee

Mix all together. Take one spoon daily

Remedy: 3

- 1 tsp apple cider vinegar

Take 1 tsp apple cider vinegar first thing in the morning on an empty stomach with half a glass of hot water.

Maintenance treatment for gout

Every day at night after supper, squeeze 1 lemon into 1 glass of warm water and sprinkle some turmeric powder into it and drink before sleeping.

Headache

Remedy :1

Headache caused through nose congestion

1 tsp full Awray (mixed) with honey & have with hot water.

Remedy: 2

- **120g ginger**
- **Vinegar**

Peel, slice and smash ginger and put black vinegar in it Soak on material and tie it to one's head and sleep with it.

Remedy: 3

Soak 5g of basil leaves in large glass of water. Let it soak. Drink the water after meals.

Remedy: 4

A handkerchief dipped in vinegar and placed on the forehead often helps to relieve the pain.

Remedy: 5

Migraine headaches

The leaves of the eucalyptus tree may be used in the treatment of migraine and other pains in the limbs due to strained muscles or after vigorous exercises.

Soften the leaves, in a tray in a hot oven. Place the heated leaves on the painful area and bandage. The treatment also relieves painful varicose veins.

Fresh mint leaves that are rubbed in the hands to release its juices may be inhaled to relieve migraine headaches.

Remedy: 6

Sneezing; Try tickling the nose with an earbud and sneeze profusely.

Heart Disease / Cholesterol

Remedy: 1

- 1 cup garlic juice
- 1 cup ginger juice
- 1 cup lemon juice
- 1 cup apple cider vinegar
- 1 cup honey

Boil all juices till it gets to 3 cups then remove from stove. When cool add the honey. Have 1 Tblsp every morning.

Remedy: 2

- ¼ cup ginger juice
- ¼ cup garlic juice
- ¼ cup green apple juice
- ¼ cup lemon juice

Boll till ¾ cup. Mix with honey and drink.

Remedy: 3

Palpitations & short breadth

- ½ tsp nut meg
- ½ tsp honey

Mix with ½ cup water and drink.

Remedy: 4

- sesame seeds
- poppy seeds
- sunflower seeds
- almonds

Grind equal amount in coffee grinder and have 1 tsp every morning.

Remedy: 5

- 11 mint leaves
- ½ tsp jeeru (cumin)
- 3 whole peppers
- 2 tsp vinegar
- 1 clove garlic

Grind together and eat

Remedy: 6

Mint tea

Boil mint leaves + 1 tsp somph (fennel) in 1 cup water, take ½ cup twice a day.

Remedy: 7

- 2 Tblsp dhania (coriander) – whole
- 1 Tblsp somph (fennel)
- 2 elachi (cardamom)
- Pinch of nutmeg (jaifal)

Grind and sift through fine sieve. Take 1 tsp after meals.

Remedy: 8

Barley Water

- 1 cup pearled barley (hull and bran removed)
- 2 litres water

Simmer the barley in a heavy-bottomed pot for about an hour or until the grains are soft and tender. Keep topping up the water and keep the lid half on. Once it is cooked, strain off the water and save the grains to eat the way you would eat rice or add to a stir-fry or soup. Keep the barley water chilled and covered in the fridge. Serve with fresh lemon juice and slice of lemon (sweeten with a touch of honey if desired) as a wonderfully refreshing drink that helps to mop up cholesterol cells. Have a glass a day of this traditional home remedy and notice the benefits!

Hiccups

Remedy: 1

- ½ tsp nutmeg (jaifal)
- ½ tsp saffron powder
- ½ tsp elachi (cardamom) powder
- honey

Combine all ingredients. Take 2 teaspoons 3 times a day.

Intestines

Remedy: 1

- 450g gulkan
- 75g ispaghul
- 100ml castor oil

Mix all the ingredients and take 1 heaped tsp at 10:30am and 3:30pm.

Indigestion

Remedy: 1

Boil 8-10 mint leaves in 1- cup of water until it turns light green, remove from heat. Add ½ tsp ground elachi. Sweeten with brown sugar or honey and take twice or thrice a day.

Remedy: 2

1 tsp vinegar in ¼ glass hot water mix together with ¼ tsp sugar. Drink as required.

Jaundice

Remedy: 1

- **7 almonds**
- **5 elachi (cardamom)**
- **2 khaarak (dried dates)**
- **hanker (sugar candy)**
- **1 tsp butter**

Leave overnight in a clay bowl (maatlu) and remove skin and pits, thereafter stamp fincly with hanker. Then mix with butter and lick it as required.

Kidney Stones

Remedy: 1

Take 2 big white radish with leaves. Wash and cut into pieces. Put into a juice extractor, add ½ cup water and extract the juice. Sift through a tea strainer and then boil it. Now sift through a cloth and let it cool. Drink at least ½ cup of radish water every morning and evening.

NB. If white radish is not available, then use red radish with the leaves.

*Avoid dairy foods, beef, tomato and achaars (pickles).

Massage Oil

Remedy: 1

- 4 litres pure India mustard oil
- 1 litre olive oil
- 250 ml eucalyptus oil
- 200g Vaseline
- 1 cup chicken fat - clean well, wash and drain all water out on a paper, melt & strain
- 125g beeswax
- 1 box camphor blocks
- 1 big tin zambuk
- 1 big bottle vicks
- 75 ml sloans liniment rub
- ¾ cup Ajmo (tymol seeds / caraway)
- 4oz (114g) Thuj (cinnamon)
- 4oz (114g) clove

- 1 Tblsp kulunji (black seeds)

Heat together 1 litre mustard oil with the ajmo, thuj, clove and kulunji. Remove from stove, then add cleaned, washed, dried and melted chicken fat and bees wax. Thereafter add all remaining ingredients. NB. Heat, DO NOT boil! - Thereafter read and blow Surah Faatiha 7 times into the pot and close the lid now ready to use as needed.

Memory

Remedy: 1

Kus-kus (poppy seeds) replaces damaged brain cells.

Remedy: 2

- 7 x badaam (almonds)

Eat every morning. Chew well

Remedy: 3

- Kus kus (poppy seeds)
- Linseed
- sunflower seeds

Grind together and have with hot milk.

Mouth sores

Remedy: 1

- 1/8th tsp sugar
- 1/8th tsp alum powder

- **1/8th tsp baking powder**

Make the above into a fine powder and mix with glycerine & English rose. Apply on the sores.

Nausea

Remedy: 1

Braise a Few elachi (cardamom) until black. Grind fine with peel and add a pinch of salt. Take ½ tsp of this with water 2-3 times a day.

Remedy: 2

Make chutney with mint leaves and elachi (cardamom), take ½ tsp 2-3 times a day.

Remedy: 3

Mix 1-2 Tblsp of lemon juice with water and drink.

Nose Bleeding

Remedy: 1

- **18g coconut fibre**
- **18g brown sugar**

Take coconut fibre and burn until almost black. Grind in coffee grinder then sift through a strainer. Mix sugar and fibre. Could be taken in 3 doses (12g each), or take 2 tsp morning and evening until all the fibre is finish. Mix in a little honey to make it easier to swallow.

Remedy: 2

2-3 drops onion juice in each nostril.

Phlegm

Remedy: 1

- **1 tsp grated ginger**
- **1-2 pieces cassia**
- **1 ¾ cup water**

Boil together until half, drink 1 hour before you sleep.

Remedy: 2

Slit a guava into 4 and sprinkle generously with black pepper. Bake it, or put it into a small pot, cover and cook on slow heat until done. Eat last thing at night while hot.

*Avoid eating lettuce, cucumber, dairy products and wheat products.

Piles

Remedy: 1

Eat beetroot.

Remedy: 2

Eat 1 guava daily for 40 days.

Pressure

Remedy: 1

- **Medium potato grated**

Squeeze and drink the water and place the grated potato On the head for 1- hour.

Remedy: 2

(Low pressure)

- Liquorice

Remedy: 3

(High Pressure)

- **1 tsp Dry Dhana (coriander)**
- **1 tsp Somph (fennel)**
- **6 Raisins**

Soak overnight in hot water and drink the next morning.

Remedy: 4

- **4-5 Hekta Sticks (drum sticks)**
- **4-5 Cups water**

Cut hekta into pieces. Boil with water until half remains. Strain. Keep in fridge. Drink ½ cup in the morning + ½ cup in the evening.

Remedy: 5

- **50g Dhana Dhal**
- **50g Somph (fennel)**
- **10g White Pepper**
- **50g Sugar**

Grind First 3 ingredients fine, then add sugar. Take 2. tsp full upon awakening + after Asr with water.

*Celery eaten daily helps to control blood pressure and cleans jaundice + uric acid.

Remedy: 6

1. Boil 1 stem parsley in 1 cup water. Drink every morning and make a fresh cup every day.
2. Soak feet in cold water.
3. Eat bananas and apples.
4. Cut out fats and salt from the diet.

Psoriasis

Avoid the following totally:

Steak, Sea—food (all types), Chocolate and Chocolate products, Sour stuff, Atchaars, all kinds of Sauces (especially sweet sour Sauce), crushed Green Chillies and Crushed Elachie (can be cooked in food whole but don't eat it), Brinjal, Milo and Hot Chocolate, no Microwave heated food, no re-heated rice and no re-heated potatoes.

- Use Rock Salt for cooking
- Drink at least 5 glasses of water during the day

Rash

Remedy: 1

- Slinger berry leaves
- 2 tsp turmeric

Slinger Berry leaves have a cooling antiseptic effect on rashes. Grind the leaves with 2 tsp turmeric and dilute in 2 litres of water. Bathe the rash affected area with this solution. Do not use soap when using the solution.

Rejuvenate

Remedy: 1

Equal parts of:
- coriander (dhania)
- ginger powder
- aniseed
- raw sugar
- water

Mix into a paste, eat 2 spoons after meals 3 times week.

Ringworms

Remedy: 1

- wild aloe
- coconut oil
- sulphur

Slit wild aloe. Rub over affected area, when dry rub paste on. Paste: mix coconut oil and sulphur.

Sprain

Remedy: 1

- 3 Tblsp brown sugar
- 3 Tblsp arad (haldi/ turmeric powder)
- one beaten egg white

Warm brown sugar and arad (haldi / turmeric powder) on stove add to it one beaten egg white. Apply on sprain. Cover with cotton wool and bandage leave for at least 24 hours.

Remedy: 2

- ¼ cup rough salt
- 1 Tblsp arad (haldi / turmeric powder)

Soak affected limb in hot water with ¼ cup rough salt and 1 Tblsp arad (haldi / turmeric powder).

Stings

Remedy: 1

For a bee, jelly fish or blue-bottle sting, dab vinegar on affected area.

Stomach Pain

Remedy: 1

- ¼ tsp B.i Soda
- Pinch of salt
- 2 tsp vinegar

Mix the above and add to ¼ glass off orange juice and drink.

Remedy: 2

1 cup of warm, honey water.

Remedy: 3

½ cup buttermilk and curry leaves. Liquidise and drink in the morning.

Strength

Remedy: 1

Linseed & sunflower seeds for strength.

Remedy: 2

1 Tblsp flaxseed oil daily.

Stroke

Remedy: 1

- 1 cup fresh garlic

Clean and cut into 4 pieces. Add garlic to 1 litre water. Mix half cup garlic water with ½ cup tap water and drink every morning.

Remedy: 2

- 2 cups onion juice
- 1 tsp heeng (asafoetida)

Mix and rub on limbs or affected area.

Throat

Remedy: 1

(Swelling of the throat)

Boil ½ tsp of crushed garlic in a cup of water. Allow to cool. When still warm, use to gargle. Mix a tsp of lime juice with a Tblsp of honey. Store in a jar and suck small quantities frequently.

Remedy: 2

(Laryngitis - inflammation of voice box)

- Cup of milk
- Pinch of turmeric powder
- Few broken pepper corn

Boil a cup of milk. Add a pinch of turmeric powder, a Few pepper corns. Drink hot every night for three nights. Will be of great benefit.

Remedy: 3

- **1 Tblsp whole wheat**
- **1 cup water**
- **salt**

Boil 1 Tblsp whole wheat in 1 cup water until water level drops to ¼ cup. Add salt and drink.

Remedy: 4

(Sore throat)

- **½ tsp B.i soda**
- **2 tsp fine salt**
- **2 tsp vinegar**
- **1 cup hot water**

Mix together and gargle

Remedy: 5

3 Tblsp boiling water, I Tblsp apple cider vinegar (gargle). Mix salt with warm water and gargle twice daily. Ideally in the morning after brushing teeth. Helps itchy and sore throat.

Remedy: 6

- **½ cup water**
- **1 tsp vinegar**

- **1 tsp honey**
- **¼ tsp fine salt**

Mix well and gargle, drink the entire mixture.

Remedy: 7

1 tsp honey stirred in a glass of hot milk.

Ulcers

Remedy: 1

The seeds of the thulsi (basil) plant which is commonly known as tukmaria may be used in milk drinks to bring relief from painful ulcers.

Infuse 1 tsp of the seeds in ½ cup water or milk. Add 1-2 blocks of sugar candy. Stir until the candy dissolves and drink at once.

Remedy: 2

(For bleeding ulcer)

Boil 50g bees wax in ½ cup milk on low heat. Scoop out melted wax with a cloth and allow to drain. Form wax into chana size pearls. Allow to dry in shaded area. Refrigerate. Swallow 2 in the morning and 2 in the evening.

Also eat pulp of the aloe plant.

Remedy: 3

Boil 8g arad (haldi / turmeric powder) dhal in 375g milk. Boil until soft as kheer (thick milk custard). Add sugar candy to sweeten and consume warm.

Vomiting & Phlegm

Remedy: 1

- **Nutmeg (jaifal) - grate on fine side.**

Mix ½ tsp nutmeg (jaifal) in 1 tsp honey, take with ¼ cup hot water.

Warts

Remedy: 1

Boil some potatoes in water. Remove the water and bathe the warts with this infusion.

Wheezing

Remedy: 1

- **1 Paan (betel) leaf**
- **1 Tsp Faake**
- **3 Sticks cinnamon**
- **3 Sticks Cloves**
- **3 Elachi (cardamom)**

Boil with ¾ cup hot water. When ¼ cup strain, add honey and drink hot.

Remedy: 2

- ½ cup water (warm)
- ½ tsp turmeric powder
- ½ tsp tsp honey (optional)

Mix well and drink 2-3 times a day. Do not drink just before and after meals.

Remedy: 3

Soak 2 onion rings in 2 tsp of honey. Leave aside for 2-3 hours or till water from onions has been extracted. Drink as often as possible.

BABIES AND MOTHERS

For Colic Babies

Remedy: 1

- 9 rose petals
- 1 Tblsp somph (fennel)
- 11 mint leaves
- 1 cup water

Boil until half. Feed to colic babies.

Remedy: 2

- 1 tsp ajmo (tymol seeds/caraway)
- 1 cup water

Mix and bring to boil. Remove and sweeten to taste. Give child to drink.

Balm to rub on chest for children with Colds

- **500ml Vaseline**
- **50g vicks**
- **20ml camphorated oil**
- **20ml olive oil**
- **20ml eucalyptus oil**

Melt Vaseline and vicks. Remove from stove and add remaining ingredients. Mix properly. Sat in airtight container.

Infants Cold

Betel leaves, heated and applied to the ribs of an infant with camphorated oil, will draw the cold and relieve pain. The leaves can also be placed on the head of the baby and covered with a bonnet. When the leaves turn dark brown or black, the cold has been drawn from the body.

*Rooibos tea often helps relieve hay fever and colic in babies.

Mixture to increase Breastmilk

- **½ cup cake flour**
- **½ cup nutty wheat**
- **½ cup ground almonds**

Braise for 20min until golden brown. When cool, add ½ cup brown sugar and 1 heaped tsp elachi (cardamom). Leave in container. Mix 1 Tblsp of mixture in 1 cup milk and drink.

Natural Home Remedies

Confinement Medication

In the 9th month of pregnancy it is recommended to swallow 1 tsp of ahario/asario with milk/coffee every morning.

After Birth

1. Every morning- swallow 1 raw egg or swallow ground bor for 5 or 7 days.

2. Warm 2 Tblsp kahyo (recipe to follow) and eat with one cup coffee.

3. Drink boiled hoowa (soowa) water in place of tap water - add tsp hoowa (soowa / anise) to 1 litre water and boil.

4. Eat hoowa (soowa / anise) sook mookh after meals to eliminate wind.

5. Have porridge in the afternoon (recipe to follow)

6. For first 5 - 7 days do not have milk

7. Bor must be filled in capsules. Take 1 capsule on alternate days. (10-15 capsules)

Kahyo

- 4 Tblsp ground almonds
- 4 Tblsp desiccated coconut
- 3 Tblsp ground sugar candy
- 2 Tblsp khus-khus (poppy seeds)
- 1 Tblsp ahario/asario
- 1 Tblsp ground pistachio

- **1 Tblsp ground charoli (chirongi nuts)**
- **1 tsp ghundar (gum) - ground**
- **125g ghor (jaggery - crude solid brown sugar)**
- **2 tsp hoonth (ginger powder)**
- **2 Tblsp salaam muslee- ground**
- **2 Tblsp panja muslee- ground**
- **4 Tblsp ground hingora (water chestnut) powder**
- **3 Tblsp ghee**
- **¼ kg ghee**

Combine first 7 ingredients in a large bowl.

In a frying pan heat 1 Tblsp ghee and roast ghundar (gum) over medium heat - allow to cool.

Break lumps of ghundar and add to the above 7 dry ingredients. Then roast the ground hingora, hoonth, gokru, panja and saalam into the ghee. Add to above ingredients.

Finally in a large pot cook ghor in ¼ kg ghee. Bring to boiling point and add all the above ingredients and cook together for a few minutes over medium heat.

Cool and store in a bottle.

N.B: If one wishes to set mixture and cut squares or diamonds, more ghor and ghee will be required to bind all ingredients together.

3 O'clock porridge masala

- 4Tblsp ground almonds
- 4Tblsp dessicated coconut
- 3Tblsp ground misry (sugar candy)
- 3Tblsp ground hingora (water chestnut)
- 1Tblsp ahario/asario
- 1Tblsp ground pista
- 1Tblsp ground charoli (chirongi nuts)
- 1tsp hoonth (ginger powder)
- Semolina
- ghor (jaggery - crude solid brown sugar)
- ghee

Mix First 8 ingredients and store as masala. To make porridge, roast 2 tsp sojee (semolina / cream of wheat) in 1 tsp ghee.

Add 2 tsp of the masala (above mentioned mixed ingredients) and 1 tsp ghor. Braise well together.

Add 1 cup water and boil. Pour in a bowl and drink

N.B. Make porridge with water in the 1st week. Thereafter use ¾ cup milk and ¼ cup water.

Hoowa (soowa/anise) Sook Mookh

- 450g hoowa (soowa / anise) - sifted and cleaned
- 250g almonds- sliced
- 2T khus-khus (poppy seeds)

- 1 tsp hanchar (black salt)
- 50g sliced coconut
- 50g shoe string coconut

Roast hoowa (soowa / anise), almonds and coconut separately on low heat in oven.

Combine all ingredients in a large dish. Mix well and store in airtight bottle. Eat approx 2 tsp after Meals.

Kwaar paak

- 6 litres milk
- 500g khaarak (dry dates)
- 500g laabu (aloe)
- 100g khus-khus (poppy seeds)
- 125g sugar candy
- 100g hingora (water chestnut) powder
- 125g almond powder
- 50g pista, ground
- 50g charoli (chirongi), ground
- 50g chaar magaj, ground
- 50g salaam muslee powder
- 1tsp elachi (cardamom) powder
- 1tsp nutmeg (jaifal) powder
- 1tsp ginger powder
- sugar to taste
- 1kg ghee

Soak khaarak overnight and mince. Boil khaarak, khus-khus(poppy seeds), milk and gel of aloe.

Leave to simmer slowly and stir frequently to prevent scorching.

When moisture dries out, put in balance of ingredients and cook over low heat and when the ghee begins to float, it is ready. Preferable to set in a tray or balls could be made.

Does not need refrigeration as this is usually made at the onset of winter as it is said to prevent colds and strengthen muscles and joints.

Methi paak

- 500g ground almonds
- 250g desiccated coconut
- 400g ghor (jaggery - crude solid brown sugar)
- 250g ground misry (sugar candy)
- 200g methi (fenugreek) powder
- 60g ground hingora (water chestnut)
- 60g ground pista
- 60g ground charoli (chirongi)
- 60g ground ghundar (gum)
- 30g gokru
- 30g ground slam muslee and panja
- 30g cleaned ahario
- 30g cleaned khus-khus (poppy and seeds)
- 750g ghee
- 50g ground ginger
- 30g ground pippar (not pepper)

- **30g ground ghantora**

Roast Ghundar in a little ghee. Cool and crush. Roast hingora, saalam, panja and ghokru in more ghee and leave aside.

In a large pot, add remaining ghee and roast methi (fenugreek) powder- then add ghor.

Cook until ghor melts, then add all other dry and roasted ingredients.

Cook for a few minutes, mixing well combining all the ingredients.

Set in a tray and cut or roll into balls and store.

N.B, Ideal for back and body aches. To be taken on alternate days in winter. Add more ghee if mixture dries.

Menstruation - For pain

- **6 peepal**
- **6g dry ginger**
- **60 black pepper**
- **6g black thill**
- **25g coconut**
- **6g old ghor (jaggery - crude solid brown sugar)**

Boil ingredients; drink 1-2 cups for 10-15 days before menses. Stop immediately on beginning of menses.

For heavy bleeding

Take 1 cup boiling water and add a few pieces of Taj (cinnamon sticks). Let it cool and drink. Rest a lot.

For weakness: during confinement and periods

- **Almonds**
- **Pista**
- **fresh coconut**

Grind together. leave in fridge. Eat with ghor (jaggery - crude solid brown sugar) once or twice a day.

Also try: Mint tea, ginger tea.

Post Natal Care

Herbal bath

Combine the leaves of the gum tree, eucalyptus and guava tree. Boil in as much natural goodness of the leaves as possible. Allow the infusion to cool slightly, but it must still be hot enough for the herbal bath to work thoroughly.

General Guidelines for Health in winter

By Hakeem Jaleel Muhammad Pandor

Stop eating foods that are cold in nature or touch.

Dress warmly especially early in the morning and at night.

Increase foods that create heat in your body. E.g. Methi paak, ginger paak, ginger tea, cinnamon tea, etc.

Exercise daily till a light perspiration is noted.

Refrain from cold foods as well as foods that are dry.

Eat foods that will increase heat, i.e. meat, spice, soups, etc.

Heavy foods can be eaten slightly more as digestion improves in winter.

Do not eat foods that are very sweet.

Dress warmly at all times, inside and outside.

Do not go outside with the body or hair wet.

Keep the feet, ears and nape covered all the times.

The body should be washed regularly so as to not block the pores which will cause harm in spring.

Use oil or cream to keep your skin moisturised.

Terminology

Aamli	tamarind
Ahario / asario	linseed
Ajmo	tymol seeds / caraway
Arad / Haldi	turmeric Powder
Awray	white pepper
Badaam	almonds
Black Thill	black sesame seeds
Bloekoem Oil	eucalyptus oil
Chaar magaj	a mixture of almonds, pumpkin seeds, cantaloupe seeds and watermelon seeds.
Charoli	chirongo nuts
Dhania	coriander
Elachi	cardamom
Faake	type of sook mook with black salt
Fudina	mint
Ghee	melted butter
Ghor	jaggery (crude solid brown sugar)
Ghundar	gum
Gokru	powder made from a certain herb
Gulkan	a sweet mixture made from rose petals

Printed in Great Britain
by Amazon